MIRACLES OF HOMEOPATHY

Super Quick Prescribing, Miraculously Fast Results: How Fact-Based Homeopathy Is Changing Lives

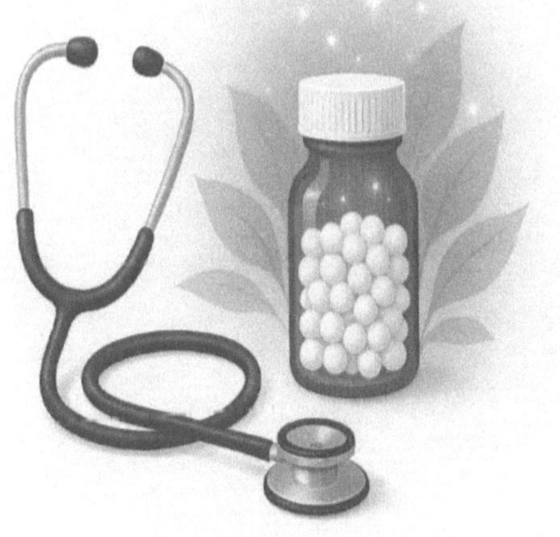

DR. JAYESH SHAH

MIRACLES

OF

HOMEOPATHY

Super-Quick Prescribing, Miraculously Fast Results – How Fact-Based Homeopathy Is Changing Lives

Dr. Jayesh Shah

DEDICATION

To my beloved mother, Late Mrs. Shobha Shah, whose unconditional love, silent strength, and eternal blessings continue to guide me every single day. Though you are no longer by my side, your presence is etched into every chapter of my life—including this one.

To my father, Mr. Hemant Shah, whose quiet sacrifices, unwavering support, and steady belief in me laid the very foundation I stand on today.

To my Mama (maternal uncle), Dr. Ghanshyam Shroff, and my Nana (maternal grandfather), the Late Dr. Ramdas Shroff, I found my calling in Homoeopathy by watching you both.

You have been my inspiration from the very beginning, and I can only hope to become a healer like both of you someday.

This book is a tribute to all of you—Some

gave me roots, some gave me wings, and all of you gave me the strength to fly.

DISCLAIMER

The information presented in this book is intended for educational and inspirational purposes only. The cases and methods described reflect the author's clinical experience and homoeopathy perspective. While every effort has been made to ensure accuracy, individual results may vary based on numerous factors, including the nature and severity of illness, patient response, and practitioner's experience.

This book is **not a substitute for professional medical advice, diagnosis, or treatment**. Readers should always seek the guidance of a qualified healthcare provider regarding any questions they may have about a medical condition or treatment plan. **Do not disregard professional medical advice or delay seeking it because of something you have read in this book.**

The methods outlined are not meant to undermine or criticise any existing school of thought within homoeopathy but to offer an alternative, fact-based approach, rooted in efficiency, clarity, and clinical outcomes. Practitioners are encouraged to apply discernment and professional judgment when considering any strategy discussed herein.

The author and publisher disclaim any liability, loss, or risk incurred directly or indirectly as a result of the application of any content of this book.

For permissions, please contact:

✉ Email: drjayeshshah07@gmail.com

A NOTE TO FELLOW HOMOEOPATHS AND STUDENTS

In this book, I have used both spellings—**"Homeopathy"** and **"Homoeopathy"**—interchangeably to ensure clarity and relatability for readers worldwide. While "Homoeopathy" is the classical spelling preferred in many parts of the world, especially in India and Europe, "Homeopathy" is more commonly used in modern international literature.

This book is written with deep respect for the art and science of Homoeopathy—and for every Homoeopath who has spent years mastering its depth. It is not a critique of tradition but an **invitation to evolve**.

What you'll find here is not theory, not fantasy, but a **system** born out of relentless clinical experience—one that aims to

simplify, **speed up**, and **strengthen** your results. If you've ever felt that lengthy case-taking is wearing out your energy or that your patients lose faith before the remedy has a chance to work, this book is for you.

I invite you to read with an **open mind and clinical curiosity**. The intention is not to divide schools of thought but to **revive the heart of Homoeopathy**: sharp observation, decisive prescribing, and life-changing results.

Let's bring back the speed, certainty, and spark that made Homoeopathy a miracle in its early days.

Welcome to a new era of healing.

— Dr. Jayesh Shah, M.D (Hom), Mumbai

ACKNOWLEDGEMENTS

Writing this book has been a journey of discovery, growth, and transformation—not only for me as a practitioner but also for my approach to healing and patient care. I am deeply grateful to everyone who has supported, inspired, and encouraged me along the way.

First and foremost, I would like to thank my **wife**, whose unwavering love, patience, and support have been my foundation throughout this process. You've always believed in my vision, even when I doubted myself, and your presence in my life continues to be my most significant source of strength. Thank you for walking this path with me, for your encouragement, and for your constant understanding.

To my **son**, who is a constant reminder of the joy of simplicity and the power of pure curiosity, thank you for inspiring me to make things more transparent and more accessible. You've taught me that learning and healing should always be a process full of wonder and discovery.

To my **father**, who taught me the values of discipline, hard work, and compassion. I carry these values with me in every patient interaction. Your wisdom and guidance have been invaluable in shaping my life and my practice. I owe so much of my success to the principles you instilled in me.

I would also like to extend my heartfelt gratitude to my **colleagues** in Homoeopathy, whose dedication to our shared profession continually challenges and motivates me. Your insights and feedback have been instrumental in shaping the ideas that make up this book. Our discussions have always pushed me to question, learn, and improve.

To my **patients**, each of you has been a source of inspiration and motivation. Your trust in me every day and the remarkable journeys we've undertaken together have been the driving force behind this book. Your courage, resilience, and belief in the healing process have given me the strength to continue learning and evolving as a practitioner.

I am also incredibly thankful for the guidance of my **teachers**. You opened my eyes to the deeper dimensions of Homoeopathy and taught me to listen—not only to the patient's symptoms but to their story, their essence. Your lessons were far more than academic; they were life-changing. To all my mentors, thank you for shaping my understanding of Homoeopathy, healing, and the world of medicine.

My heartfelt thanks to **Dr. Pooja Bharadwaj** for penning the foreword to this book. Her presence in my journey has been nothing short of a blessing. All the psychiatric cases from my OPD are confidently entrusted to her capable hands— not just because of her clinical expertise, but because of her deep compassion and unmatched diagnostic acumen. She sees what many miss and heals where many struggle. Her unwavering support, sharp insights, and quiet strength have added immense value to my practice and to this book. Thank you, Dr.

Pooja, for standing by me and for believing in this work.

Finally, a special mention goes to everyone who has shared their story, whether as a patient, a peer, or a critic. Your experiences and reflections have contributed to writing this book in ways I never anticipated. This book is not just my work; it is a collective effort—a mosaic of ideas, stories, and feedback I have had the privilege to learn from.

Thank you all, from the bottom of my heart.

Dr. Jayesh Shah

FOREWORD

When Dr. Jayesh first shared the idea behind this book with me, I knew it wouldn't be just another clinical case collection. I knew it would carry his fire—his refusal to blindly follow protocols, his commitment to facts, and his obsession with results. And now, as I hold the final manuscript in my hands, I can say with certainty—it is so much more.

This book is quite a revolution. It shakes the very foundation of how we approach cases, especially in Homoeopathy, where we are often taught to dig deep into layers upon layers of emotions, dreams, and traumas. Dr. Jayesh turns the spotlight back to the obvious—the presenting symptoms, the visible patterns, the spoken words, and the body language.

What stands out most is the simplicity with which he works—and yet, the miracles he achieves. Cases that were dismissed as hopeless... conditions that were thought to be incurable… were turned around not by two-to-three-hour marathon case-takings, but by razor-sharp observation, unshakeable clarity, and bold, honest prescribing—often within just a few minutes.

This book is a gift—not just to homeopaths but to every healer who wants to rediscover the joy of watching someone walk back into life through accurate, compassionate, and quick care. It is not a shortcut—it is a straight path. And if you follow it with an open heart and sharp mind, it will change your practice.

Dr. Jayesh, you've not only documented the power of Homoeopathy—you've made it impossible for us to ignore it.

With admiration,

Dr. Pooja R Pandey

MD Homoeopathic Psychiatrist

TABLE OF CONTENTS

CHAPTER 1

Homoeopathy in the Modern World – Why Speed and Reliability Are Crucial for Competing with Modern Medicine

It was during the early days of my practice when I first encountered a moment that shook me to my core. A middle-aged man, Mr. Sharma, had visited me for chronic acidity. His symptoms were classic—burning pain in the stomach, bloating, and occasional regurgitation. I listened patiently, carefully noting the details, and assured him that Homoeopathy would help. After prescribing a well-matched remedy, I scheduled a follow-up for next week.

But he never returned.

A few weeks later, I happened to run into him outside a mall. He looked at me with an awkward smile and said, ***"Doctor, Homoeopathy takes time... so I consulted another doctor....I wanted quick relief..."***

That brief conversation with Mr. Sharma exposed a deep and uncomfortable truth: the widespread perception that Homoeopathy is slow is far from the truth. In today's fast-paced world, this misconception needs to change.

I still remember trying to convince him. I spoke about the depth of Homoeopathy, its long-term benefits, and how it treats the root cause. But he nodded with polite disinterest, and I realised I was trying too hard. My words were falling flat, not because they were wrong, but because the world outside doesn't wait for philosophies.

If I have to explain Homoeopathy's strength repeatedly to every patient, the essence gets diluted. **Truth is not something to be begged for—it is something to be discovered.** And discovery only happens when people see results with their own eyes, not through long monologues from a hopeful doctor.

A champion athlete never spends his energy convincing the world that he is fast, strong and efficient. He doesn't chase people to prove his worth. **The world sees it when he runs or plays. The stopwatch speaks. The scoreboard speaks. His performance is the proof.** But if an athlete finds himself constantly trying to *explain* his speed and justify his strength, then something is wrong. Either he's not performing at his best, or he's in the wrong arena. **Excellence doesn't need marketing—it needs visibility.**

The same applies to Homoeopathy.

If I, as a Homoeopath, have to repeatedly tell each patient that Homoeopathy works… that it's powerful, precise, and effective… then something is off. **The truth of any system should be self-evident in its results.** A patient should feel the shift, the relief, and the transformation much quicker than they expect—and *then* they will believe.

That's the vision I am committed to: building a practice where performance speaks louder than explanations and results silence doubts. Homoeopathy doesn't need to be sold—it simply needs to be witnessed.

And that's the journey you'll enter through this book's pages.

The Shift That Changed Everything

From that day onwards, something shifted in me. I wasn't just a Homoeopath anymore—I became an observer. I started to gather facts and look closely at our system's cracks. Why don't people believe in Homoeopathy the way they do in other systems of medicine? Why does it often remain their second, third or last choice?

I didn't have to look far.

I saw the first crack in the form of long, tiring case-takings—2 to 3 hours of deep-dive sessions where the patient is expected to relive every emotion and memory, sometimes elaborating and probing unnecessary details. All this while they sit there in pain, distress and stress, hoping for relief. **We forget to value the patient's time and suffering.** Think from the patient's perspective: if someone makes you wait for 3 hours in the waiting area and then takes your case for another 3 hours—*that too when you're in pain or discomfort*—how would you feel? And even after all that, there's no guarantee when the medicine will start working. Then the doctor asks you to come back after 15 days. Would you go there again?

While other systems of medicine are constantly evolving to minimise patient wait times and deliver faster results, Homoeopathy is often found indulging in elaborate, time-consuming case-taking in the name of depth.

- **Surgeons** are constantly working to minimize surgery time and hospital stays. Many procedures are now done as **day-care surgeries**—

patients are discharged the same day.

- **Dentists** are using **3D printing and CAD/CAM technology** to offer same-day crowns and implants, reducing what used to take weeks into just one visit.

- **Physiotherapists** are integrating **advanced machines, taping techniques, and focused therapy protocols** to accelerate recovery time and reduce the number of sessions.

- **Radiologists** use digital reporting and AI-assisted scans to provide instant access to test results, saving both doctors' and patients' time.

At a time when the entire medical world is innovating to **save the patient's time, energy, and effort**, Homoeopathy is, ironically, moving in the opposite direction—**searching for ways to stretch consultations in the name of depth**, often mistaking length for insight.

Then comes the *method of prescribing*—"Give one dose and wait for 15 days." Really? **If it's your son/daughter crying in pain, will you wait for 15 days hoping something will happen?** I have a doctor friend... When his wife had a migraine, he asked her about the symptoms in just 2 minutes, quickly decided which medicine to give and gave her that medicine every half hour. She recovered completely within 2 hours (100% improvement). But if a similar case comes to his OPD, he takes a 2-3 hour-long case and provides a " deep acting" medicine... and asks the patient to come back after 15 days. The patient improves by 30% in 15 days.

And finally, perhaps the most damaging of all, I saw it in the lack of self-belief among Homoeopaths.

How often have we heard Homoeopaths themselves say:-

"It will take time.",

"You'll have to be patient.",

"Let's wait and watch...Homoeopathy is slow"

These words don't inspire trust. They signal hesitation. They tell the patient, *"Even I'm not sure."* And if the doctor isn't convinced, how can the patient ever be?

That was the wake-up call. From that moment, I knew **it was time for a change.**

Homoeopathy is not weak—It's just that some of the newer approaches, which seem more like fantasy, have diverted our attention from pure symptom-based and fact-based Homoeopathy. We've come to believe that the more time we spend on a case, the better our prescription will be.

Remember, a skilled expert only taps the surface, and he quickly understands whether gold, iron, or glass is beneath it. He will know it by the surface's sound when he taps it. He doesn't need to dig deep to know what lies underneath.

You, too, can become the kind of expert

who, with just a few fact-based questions, a sharp eye, and focused attention, can find in minutes what someone might take hours to uncover.

This book will help you get there.

CHAPTER 2

The Problem with Traditional Case-Taking – The Inefficiency of 2-3 Hour Marathon Sessions

For years, Homoeopathy has been synonymous with lengthy, exhaustive consultations. Practitioners spend two to three hours listening to a patient's life history, exploring their deepest emotions, childhood traumas, and even dreams. The belief is that the more details we gather, the better the remedy selection. But is this necessary?

Why Long Case-Taking is a Problem

Reason 1: Patients Want Quick Relief,

Not a Therapy Session

Modern patients do not have the patience for marathon consultations. Unlike the 18th and 19th centuries, when people had the time to narrate their life stories, today's patients are accustomed to quick medical visits. They visit a doctor because they want **solutions, not lengthy discussions.**

Consider this: if a patient has an acute headache or severe gastritis, will they be willing to sit for three hours and recall their childhood fears? **No.** They will walk out and find a quicker solution, often turning to Allopathy, which provides immediate relief.

One of the biggest traps in modern Homoeopathic practice is the tendency to overcomplicate even the simplest cases. This practice often begins with good intentions—the Homoeopath wants to understand the patient deeply, to go beyond the surface, to "see the person behind the disease." But in this pursuit, something crucial is lost: clarity.

Many doctors today are trained to keep

digging, especially into the mental and emotional realms. They're taught that the *"real remedy"* lies not in the patient's symptoms, but in their "deep inner world". While this may sound noble and even poetic, the reality in the clinic can be far from it.

As the doctor asks more questions, many of which seem unrelated to the chief complaint, the patient begins to sense what the doctor is fishing for. And that's where the real problem begins.

To fit the doctor's narrative and not appear "too normal" or "uninteresting," the patient starts to construct stories. Not because they want to lie, but because they want to be understood. They want to seem unique. They want to give the doctor something valuable to work with.

And so, unconsciously or consciously, the patient begins to present themselves as victims of their circumstances, their family, society, or fate. They speak in dramatic metaphors and describe events with theatrical flair. Suddenly, their life becomes a series of emotional storms and personal betrayals, and the rest of the world becomes the villain.

The doctor, deeply engrossed in the session, starts noting down these so-called "unique mentals." They feel proud to have uncovered something *deep* and *individualized*. The session may last for an hour, two hours, or sometimes even more. By the end, the doctor is satisfied and convinced they have found the "core delusion" or the "central disturbance."

But what has really happened? The doctor was led on a rabbit hunt through the jungle of the patient's imagination. What was a straightforward case of acidity, headache, or joint pain has now become a psychological thriller with no solid ground. And worse, no remedy is rooted in observable, factual, physical data.

This is where modern Homoeopathy often fails.

Because in trying to intellectualise every case, we forget that healing is not an art of dramatic stories. It's a science of observation, clarity, and practical action. We must never forget:

"A case is not deep because it is emotional. A case is deep when it is clear."

We don't need to turn every patient into a novel. Sometimes, the remedy is right there—in the symptoms, in the modalities, in the physicals—in plain sight. Sometimes, in search of " depth", we miss the diamond lying on the surface, right in front of us.

The patient came for relief. Not for a personality excavation.

We must ask ourselves, "Are we solving the case or *admiring our detective work?* "

Let us return to simplicity, not out of laziness, but out of respect for the patient's time, truth, and trust.

Reason 2: Long Case-Taking Does Not

Guarantee Better Accuracy

Some Homoeopaths believe that the more they listen, the better they understand the patient. However, **too much information can dilute the most important symptoms.** The reality is that patients often share **irrelevant** details, such as:

- What they dreamed of last week
- How they felt when they were 10 years old
- Random fears that may or may not be related to their condition.

I remember a patient who came with severe headaches—bursting pain at 11 a.m., worse from sun and noise, better with pressure. Clear modalities, clear timeline.

But instead of trusting these facts, the previous doctor had spent hours probing her childhood trauma and relationship patterns. The prescription was missed. The pain remained.

When I prescribed Natrum muriaticum

200, based on the exact modalities, the fact that she came to me in peak summer season, when sun exposure headaches are common, her headache disappeared within 2 hours.

In nearly 90% of headache cases that walk into your clinic during the summer, the remedies often point toward Natrum muriaticum or Glonoine, because these patients are aggravated by heat and sun. If their headaches worsened due to the cold, they wouldn't be coming in during April, May, or June—they'd show up in winter instead.

The very season in which the patient seeks help is a powerful diagnostic clue. When someone who remains cheerful all through winter suddenly comes to you at the first hint of summer heat, their timing alone begins to tell a story. It reflects when their suffering intensifies. It reflects what is intolerable for them. It gives you a ready-made and obvious modality which you don't need to excavate. It presented itself.

But most practitioners ignore this. They

dive into emotions and life stories, while the real trigger—the sun beating down and the hot weather—sits ignored on the surface.

Start looking at the season as a part of the totality. It's a simple fact, hiding in plain sight. And when you notice it, you'll begin to see what others miss.

Reason 3: Seeing Fewer Patients Forces High Consultation Fees, Thereby Making Homoeopathy Unaffordable For Many

A Homoeopath who spends three hours per patient can **only see 3-4 patients daily**. This creates two significant problems:

1. It limits the number of people who can benefit from Homoeopathy.
2. It forces the doctor to charge high fees to compensate for the low patient volume.

For example, if a Homoeopath wants to earn **₹1,00,000 per month** but can only see

80-100 patients per month due to long case-taking sessions, they are forced to charge around **₹1,000 - ₹1,200 per consultation** to sustain their practice. Some Homoeopaths even charge **₹2000-4000 per consultation in big cities.** It becomes almost impossible for **middle-class** families to afford them, especially when 2-3 members of the same family need medical attention at the same time.

Compare this to a Homoeopath who sees **10-15 patients daily** using a **faster, fact-based approach.** They can charge **₹300-₹500 per consultation** and still earn the same or even more.

The **first** Homoeopath is limited in reach and caters only to an **elite, high-income group**.

The **second** Homoeopath makes Homoeopathy **affordable for middle-class and lower-income families**, ensuring that more people benefit from it.

The biggest irony is that **Homoeopathy is**

supposed to be a common man's medicine, yet these lengthy, inefficient consultations have made it more of a luxury.

Instead of becoming a mainstream, affordable healthcare option, Homoeopathy is slowly becoming an **exclusive, high-cost service.** This will make it very difficult for it to be everyone's first choice.

Reason 4. The Myth That Homoeopathy Needs Months and Years to Work

Some argue that lengthy case-taking is necessary because Homoeopathy takes time to act. This is **a myth.**

If the correct remedy is given, acute cases can show results in minutes or hours. If prescribed with precision, chronic cases, too, can show significant improvement within days.

Homoeopathy works fast **when the remedy selection is precise and symptom-**

based. The problem is not the medicine—it's the **time wasted on unnecessary details.**

The Solution: Fast, Fact-Based Case-Taking

Instead of focusing on irrelevant emotional narratives, Homoeopathy should rely on transparent, objective, and reproducible symptoms.

- What are the **chief complaints** and their ODP (Onset, duration and Progress)?
- What are the **objective symptoms?** (physical signs, appearance of the lesion, appearance in general, lab results, pathology)
- What are the **modalities**? (What makes it better or worse?)
- What is the general state of the patient? (energy, sleep, appetite)

Subsequent chapters will discuss my exact

case-taking method. Remember that a **15-minute focused consultation** can yield better results than a **3-hour deep dive into emotions and dreams.**

Conclusion: Faster Case-Taking, Better Homoeopathy

The inefficiency of marathon sessions is one of the biggest reasons why Homoeopathy struggles to compete with modern medicine. By **shortening consultation time, focusing on facts, and prescribing efficiently,** we can:

- See and help more patients daily
- Get faster results
- Make Homoeopathy a first-choice system instead of a last resort
- Make it **affordable and accessible** to the common man

The time has come to **redefine Homoeopathy**—not by changing its core principles but by **eliminating methods that slow it down.**

CHAPTER 3

The Power of Fact-Based Prescribing

"When Clarity meets precision, miracles happen"- Unknown

In a world where data drives decision-making, from aviation to medicine, Homoeopathy must evolve beyond the fog of speculation and embrace the light of facts.

Fact-based prescribing doesn't mean abandoning our philosophy and our core principles. It means applying it with clarity. It's about anchoring ourselves in what the patient is actually experiencing, not what we or the patient imagine.

Gone are the days when a Homoeopath had to play psychologist, therapist, and philosopher in one session. We truly need a sharp eye for observable, repeatable, and confirmable symptoms.

The Beauty of What Is Obvious

A patient with asthma aggravated by dust, cold air, and exertion doesn't need to be asked how he felt when his father scolded him at age 9. Right in front of you, the facts are speaking. You notice she keeps moving her hands and legs—classic restlessness. The remedy is almost waving at you: **Arsenicum album**. Yet, many Homoeopaths miss this because their minds are busy chasing an elusive "peculiar mental symptom," hoping to uncover some "buried trauma", some fancy " delusion". In doing so, they overlook the obvious. The body is already telling the story—**you need to stop over-listening and start observing.**

Modalities never lie; Memories often do.

When a patient says, "My pain gets worse on bending forward," you have a fact. But when he says, "I feel like my heart is broken every morning," you're already in the fog.

In Homoeopathy, modalities—those specific conditions that make a symptom better or worse—are like the body's native language: clear, consistent, and rooted in observation. They bypass the stories we tell ourselves, the emotional narratives that can change with time, memory, or mood.

Take Magnesia phosphoricum: When the patient says, "I have abdominal cramps that ease with warmth or pressure," you don't need to hear about their exam anxiety from fifth grade.

Or Rhus tox: "I feel stiff in the morning, but as I keep moving, it gets better." That one modality can guide you more confidently than twenty minutes of trying to decode childhood guilt.

Or Bryonia: "Even the slightest movement worsens my pain. I just want to lie still." That single line is your compass.

Modalities are constant. A person might forget what triggered their emotional breakdown last year, but they will not forget that cold water aggravates their throat pain or that their headache vanishes when they lie in a dark, quiet room.

Even in psychiatric cases—yes, even there—modalities show up. A patient with anxiety may say, "My palpitations get worse after eating," or "I feel breathless when I lie flat." These are not random details—they're doors to the remedy.

Meanwhile, the moment we slip too far into unverified mental interpretations—like "he feels betrayed by society," or "she is emotionally frozen due to childhood trauma"—we risk entering a maze with no exit. The danger? We may prescribe on fiction, not fact.

Note: When in doubt, return to the modalities. They won't embellish, they won't exaggerate—they just quietly point to the remedy.

Don't chase shadows in a fog when the body is holding a torch.

Let's understand this better with the help of a clinical case where a remedy based on mental symptoms failed, but a modality-based approach led to quick recovery:

Patient: A 55-year-old man with severe joint pain, especially in his knees and shoulders.

Without asking him about the modalities, the previous Homoeopath jumped directly into deep mental exploration. He unearthed suppressed anger, years of frustration and indignation at work. He prescribed Staphysagria 200. The patient was not better even after 2 months.

The Doctor increased the dose to 1m, and even that failed to act.

Frustrated, the Doctor took the case again. This time, he found out that the patient had not given the history of his mother's death and how it affected him. The doctor scolded the patient for not giving a proper case history the first time and, this time, considering chronic grief as the centre point, gave Natrum

Mur 200.

Result: The patient's condition worsened to the extent that he lost all faith in Homoeopathy.

The patient then came to me when one of my other patients forced him to show me at least once.

I stressed the modalities. Below is how the conversation went :

"When does the pain worsen?"

"With any movement."

"What makes it better?"

"If I lie absolutely still and rest the joint."

"Anything else that you could think of which increases or decreases the pain?"

"Yes, Doctor, pressing makes it worse. I tried a home massage to get some relief, but it worsened my state"

The picture was now loud and clear—**Bryonia alba.**

Prescription: Bryonia Alba 30, tds for 3 days.

Follow-up 3 days later: *"Much better, Doctor. I slept peacefully. I'm able to sit and work now without needing a painkiller. The pain is almost 95% better."*

***Follow-up* after 15 days:** *"I'm not in pain now. Doctor, I can't believe Homoeopathy acts so fast"*

The Takeaway: Not once did the patient say *"I feel emotionally hurt,.* But his body clearly said: *"Don't move me."*

Bryonia didn't come from a mental maze. It walked in clearly through the door of modalities—pain aggravated by motion, relieved by rest.

In cases like these, stories distract, but **modalities direct.**

CASE OF INFLATED MENTALS

Let us see one more case.

A few years ago, a young female doctor friend of mine, just out of her post-graduation, shared an interesting case with me. A 48-year-old male patient walked into her clinic with an air of confidence and charisma. He was sharply dressed, well-spoken, and had this calm, philosophical tone as he began describing his issue: **constipation**. But instead of sticking to the facts, he started giving her a full-blown monologue.

"I don't think it's just physical," he told her. *"It's more existential. I hold on to things—emotions, control, disappointments. Maybe that's why my body can't let go either."*

He painted a picture of himself as a deep thinker, misunderstood, someone who felt things intensely but rarely expressed them. He spoke of childhood betrayals, perfectionism, and his dislike for emotional messiness.

Being new and a bit impressionable, my friend took all this at face value. She felt like she was sitting with a rare, complex, emotional personality. So, she prescribed a deep-acting constitutional remedy, Carcinosin 1m, that she thought fit the mental picture he had presented.

A week later, the patient returned. His constipation was unchanged. He smiled and said, *"I am not better, but I know Homoeopathy takes time, and my body is tough to treat, so small doses don't affect me much"* He sounded like he was trying to impress her again. This time, my friend decided to step back from the drama and called him the next day.

That evening, she called me on the phone, and I suggested she ask the questions in the following way. When the patient came the next day, she was clear on what to ask.

"When exactly is your constipation

worse?" she asked.

"*In the mornings,*" he replied, "*I get the urge, but nothing comes out. I sit for 15-20 minutes. I try to defecate multiple times, but pass small quantities every time. After multiple attempts in the morning, I get frustrated and angry. And if I try too hard, I end up with a headache. It ruins my mood for the entire day.*"

"**Anything else related to your constipation**?" she asked.

He said, "Yes, I have to strain a lot, even to pass those small quantities of stool."

Now unsure about the initial prescription, she called me to ask what remedy would fit best. I told her, "*Forget the philosophy for a minute. Just focus on the facts*"

That's when it clicked for her. Everything about the case screamed **Nux Vomica**—the ineffectual urging, the straining, the irritability, the morning aggravation, and the overall temperament.

She gave him a dose of Nux Vomica 200, and within a few days, the patient reported normal, easy stools. His mood had improved, too. He wasn't trying to act deep or poetic anymore—he was just relieved.

Later that evening, she called me again. Still puzzled, she asked, "*But why didn't you consider Bryonia? He did seem quite industrious, mentally organised, even business-like.*"

I smiled. "*You're going down the same confusing path again,*" I said gently. "*You're giving weight to a mental picture that the patient crafted to impress you. But the facts— they were screaming for attention.*"

I reminded her that Nux Vomica has ineffectual urging. The patient keeps going to the toilet repeatedly, passing little each time. That's why the patient goes for defecation multiple times.

On the other hand, Bryonia has dryness of all the mucous membranes. The person doesn't even feel the desire to go. When he does, it's once in two or three days. Because the passage is too dry, a long, dry and hard stool forms. In Nux Vomica, small, frequent stool passes due to ineffectual urging.

She was quiet for a moment. Then said, "*I see it now.*"

"*If you pay attention,*" I said, "*the facts tell you everything. The truth doesn't hide—it just gets buried under too many questions.*"

We laughed about it later. I told her, "***The mind can perform, but the gut doesn't lie.***" She agreed. That case taught her one of the most important lessons early in her practice—don't get hypnotised by the mental show. Trust the body's language

In the world of Homoeopathy, facts are not just data—they're the voice of the disease itself. When we shift our attention from abstract narratives to concrete modalities, something magical happens—**clarity emerges**. You begin to see what others miss. No more guessing games, no more chasing shadows. The real miracle of

Homoeopathy lies not in mystical prescriptions, but in the precision of listening to the body's language. **Prescribe what you can prove. Trust what you see.** That's where the real power lies.

CHAPTER 4

Imagination vs. Facts – The Biggest Mistake You Are Making in Your Clinics

Have you ever noticed how a single thought, seemingly harmless, can pull you into an emotional quicksand by the end of the day?

Let's take a simple example.

You wake up. It's a normal morning.

Then, your phone rings once and goes silent.
You check. It's a missed call. No message.
No follow-up.

That's when it begins.

Your mind whispers: *"Who was it? Why*

didn't they call again?"

Then, the anxiety creeps in.

"Last time something like this happened, it was from my kid's school... he had fallen sick. What if it's something urgent again?"

A knot forms in your stomach. You suddenly feel guilty:

"Am I being careless as a parent? Why didn't I pick up immediately?"

Then, the self-blame gains speed.

"I've been missing a lot of things lately... I skipped the gym three times last week. I didn't reply to that important email. I still haven't followed up on Dad's health check-up."

The spiral tightens.

From a single missed call, your mind has crafted a narrative in which you're irresponsible, failing at multiple roles, and on the verge of losing control. **Nothing *actually* happened, but emotionally, you've lived a crisis.**

That's the dangerous power of imagination. It feeds on assumptions, half-memories, and emotional residue. It builds castles in the air—but sometimes, they're made of fear, not hope.

Now, apply this to the clinic.

A patient walks in. You ask one emotionally loaded question.

And the spiral begins.

They remember something their uncle said 20 years ago.

Then connect it to how they felt after failing an exam. Then begin to imagine how that created their current "insecurity."

Before long, they themselves are convinced that their eczema is psychosomatic, caused by unresolved grief from adolescence.

The worst part? Many doctors take this path with them, becoming silent partners in the journey. Instead of gently opening the patient's eyes to reality, they drift into the patient's imagined world, lost in the illusion they were meant to dispel.

They call it **"going deep,"** when in fact, it's just **going vague**.

They chase imagined emotions and symbolic interpretations— While the *real*, *observable*, *tangible* symptoms sit untouched like :

"It burns when he scratches it."

"It gets worse after bathing."

"The skin is red, cracked, and itchy at night."

This is the great divergence—the fork at which your practice either stays rooted in facts or floats away into a fog of **subjective imagination**.

And only one of those paths leads to tangible results.

Why Only in Homoeopathy?

In every other walk of life, we demand facts. We don't entertain vague promises or run after imagination.

When you're building a house, would you trust a builder who simply describes a grand vision without showing a single flat or apartment he's built before? Of course not. You'd want a site visit, proof of previous projects, customer feedback, and **facts** that back his claims.

Or take investing—whether it's in stocks or starting a business. We spend hours poring over numbers, asking, "Is this company profitable? What's the debt ratio? Who are the founders?" We look at annual reports, balance sheets, and past performance. No one puts money into a company that just says, *"We believe we'll do well"*. You will say, " *Show us the proof, the hard data, the balance sheet, so that we can believe in your company's potential"*.

Even in relationships, we value consistent actions over dreamy words. You won't trust someone who keeps promising change but never follows through.

So then, **why only in Homoeopathy—where your health, your peace, and even your life are at stake—do we often throw away this need for certainty? And instead chase after whims, fantasies, and castles in the air?**

Why do some practitioners—and even patients—leave the solid ground of facts and climb the slippery slope of imagined trauma, invented grief, and speculative narratives?

Your body doesn't lie. It shows you the facts every day through modalities, patterns, sensations, and objective symptoms. So, when choosing a remedy, don't abandon that clarity. Hold on to it with the exact tight grip you'd have when investing your life savings.

- "You wouldn't build a house on an architect's *imagination* without seeing any blueprint or sample flat.
- You wouldn't invest in a company just because the founder says, 'We imagine being the next big thing.'
- You wouldn't trust a partner who keeps saying they'll change, without any real change.

Then why, in Homoeopathy—where your body, your mind, and your health are on the line—do you leave the facts behind and dive into imagination?

Always remember, you're not just healing a condition—you're building health. And like every solid house, it needs a **foundation built on facts.**

CHAPTER 5

Individualistic Approach Vs Specific Approach

We, as a system of healing, are lagging behind—not because we lack depth, but because we sometimes go *too deep* in the wrong direction. The obsession with "individualisation" has reached a point where many Homoeopaths are more interested in unearthing the "peculiar symptoms", the " Man behind the disease", that they forget that even the common symptoms, when present, clearly point to the " **Man behind the disease**". In our desperate quest to find what makes a patient "unique," we forget that he didn't come to us to have his personality analysed—he came to be relieved from suffering.

I've seen Homoeopaths glowing with pride after charting out an elaborate list of mental rubrics. They feel as if they've unearthed a hidden jewel from the ocean, forgetting that what the patient really needs is a **solution**, not a **treasure map**. They place these imaginative mental symptoms above concrete, observable facts—modalities, locations, sensations, and physical generals.

It is like a fireman arriving at the scene of a burning house. Instead of putting out the fire, he starts analysing the building's architectural style. Yes, the structure might be interesting, but that's not what needs immediate attention.

By giving unnecessary weight to speculative emotional states, we risk turning our prescriptions into a guessing game. Real healing happens when we return to what is *reliable*—what can be seen, touched, and confirmed. Facts don't lie. Modalities don't lie. The body speaks its truth through symptoms, not through a dramatic retelling of inner trauma that may or may not even be accurate.

If true individuality exists in a case, it will shine on its own—you won't have to play detective in the dark. When a patient repeatedly mentions that *every complaint feels better by lying on the painful side* and *worse from any noise or light*, **Natrum mur** stands up and salutes without needing a deep psychoanalysis.

Or take a patient who complains of *pains that are tearing and shifting from one joint to another, worse from rest and cold, and better by motion*—you don't need to dive into his childhood trauma to recognise **Rhus tox.**

Individuality isn't a buried treasure you need to dig ten feet down to find; it's more like a lighthouse guiding you, provided your eyes are open to see it. The irony is, the more you dig for *hidden emotions*, the more you risk burying the truth that's already lying on the surface.

In fact, the remedies with the strongest personality patterns—like Nux vomica's irritability or Arsenicum's restlessness and insecurity—never hide in metaphors or abstract memories. They walk into the clinic wearing a name tag. And when you try to ignore this clarity and keep asking, *"But how did you feel when your uncle ignored you at age 12?"*, you miss what the case practically screams. The truth is, individuality doesn't whisper from the shadows—it speaks from the centre, loud and clear.

Individuality in Homoeopathy is like a face in a crowd—it stands out if it truly belongs. But if you keep forcing it, inventing stories, and digging endlessly, maybe it's not there. The more you chase imagination, the more likely you are to lose touch with reality

Don't be like a warrior who is hunting a phantom in the jungle—no matter how hard you try, you will end up with twigs and scratches.

Belicve me, most of the remedies will be apparent in the first few minutes of the consultation if you focus on the facts and observe closely.

You don't need rocket science for that; just an open sensory system (Eyes, ears, nose, etc.), a mindset that it's possible, and a basic knowledge of Materia Medica. That's it.

By going with the facts, you will do far better than those wandering through a maze of psychological guesswork, **searching for a key in a room that was never locked.**

The Power of Specific Fact-Based Prescription

Let us now see some cases where the remedy shouted itself in the first few minutes of consultation. But before you read on, just pay attention to the cases as if they had come to your clinic and try to find out the remedy yourself. You will notice that if you, too, focus on the facts instead of going unnecessarily deeper every time, you will find the remedy in minutes, if not seconds. So, let's see some cases:

CASE NO 1: CHRONIC BRONCHITIS

A 50-year-old man walked slowly and cautiously into the clinic as if every movement came with a price. His face was slightly pale, and his brows were furrowed in pain. He gently supported his chest with one hand, clearly guarding the area as he settled stiffly into the chair.

"*It hurts every time I breathe,*" he said, pausing to catch his breath. "*If I move... even talk... it worsens. I just want to lie down and not be disturbed. I have seen multiple doctors over the past month; they have diagnosed it as Bronchitis, but none of them were able to give me relief*" His voice carried a faint irritability, not toward the doctor but toward the very discomfort that gripped him.

Even before the case could proceed further, the remedy had nearly written itself on the walls.

Every sentence, every gesture pointed unmistakably toward **Bryonia**:

— The **pain is aggravated by motion** in any form, even the slightest shifting in posture.

— The **desire to lie completely still**, as if the

body knew that movement would only amplify suffering.

— The **irritability** is not from psychological conflict but from the overwhelming physical distress.

Here, one could easily begin a detailed inquiry into whether his boss had overloaded him at work, whether he had been suppressing frustration, or if there had been recent emotional tension at home. But that would have been a detour into imagination.

The truth was right there: **movement aggravates, rest relieves**. The body had chosen its own defence mechanism—**immobility**—and was screaming for a remedy that resonated with that state.

In this case, **Bryonia didn't just whisper. It shouted.** No probing needed. No mental acrobatics. Just **listening to the body's story**—spoken through facts, not fantasies.

CASE NO 2
DYSMENORRHOEA

A young woman in her mid-twenties entered my clinic. Even before sitting before me, she did something that caught my attention: She gently pushed the consultation chamber's door wide open.

She said in a soft tone " *Sorry doctor, I hope you don't mind me keeping it open, I feel suffocated in close chambers, keeping it open will allow fresh air to come inside*".

That was the first clue.

She then went on to describe her painful menses. She had undergone sonography, but no visible abnormality was found. The periods were crampy, exhaustive and profuse.

I asked her about the exact location of the pain, and she said, " *It's not fixed, doctor, it keeps changing. Sometimes lower back, sometimes lower abdomen, sometimes thighs, even the severity keeps changing from mild to moderate to severe*"

As I was going through her Sonography reports and her other investigations, I found out that she has had UTIS (Urinary Tract infections) 3 times in the last 2 months and took antibiotics for the same.

I asked her a direct question: "*UTIS (Urinary Tract Infections) so many times in 2 months? How much is your water intake?*"

She said, " *Doctor, I don't feel like drinking water. Even if the bottle is in front of me, I avoid drinking from it.*"

The remedy was shouting itself loud and clear by now.

Thirstlessness. Desire for open air. Changeable symptoms. Her mild nature --- all pointing towards **Pulsatilla.**

Pulsatilla was not hiding in the depths of some traumatic childhood memory or unresolved emotional complex. **It was right there, in the opening symptoms, in the**

modalities and her way of carrying herself.

In Homoeopathy, the truth often walks in before the patient even sits down. It speaks through posture, breath, gestures, tones, and the most practical of needs. The art of prescribing isn't about unravelling cryptic emotional puzzles hidden in forgotten corners of the mind—it's about listening with clarity, observing with honesty, and honouring **the facts**.

When you tune into what the body and behaviour plainly say, remedies begin to select themselves. No mental gymnastics, no philosophical rabbit holes—just grounded, **fact-based prescribing** that delivers results. Let others get lost in the fog of fantasy if they wish; you, dear reader, now know where the light is—and it shines brightly on the **undeniable truth of symptoms** that speak when you are willing to listen.

CHAPTER-6

Real-Life Miracles: No 3-Hour Marathons, Straightforward Prescriptions, Stunning Results

In an age where long-drawn case-taking is often glorified as the pinnacle of Homoeopathic practice, what often gets lost is the simplicity and elegance of clear, fact-based prescribing.

In my clinic, I've witnessed jaw-dropping recoveries—cases where even seasoned doctors had given up hope—transformed not by emotional deep dives or philosophical exploration but by sharp, focused observation and understanding of modalities.

These were not 3-hour marathons filled with intellectual somersaults. These were 5 to 10-minute consults where the remedy didn't whisper—it roared. The body spoke. The facts aligned. And the cure followed.

CASE NO 1: BLACK HAIRY TONGUE
(LINGUA VILLOSA NIGRA)

She walked in with a **thick black patch growing on her tongue**, spreading like a carpet of soot. Most people suspected it to be fungal; others feared something worse.

She was told to go for antifungal mouthwashes, swabs, biopsies, and even blood tests to rule out cancer. She was unable to eat or drink, and her condition seemed to be worsening day by day.

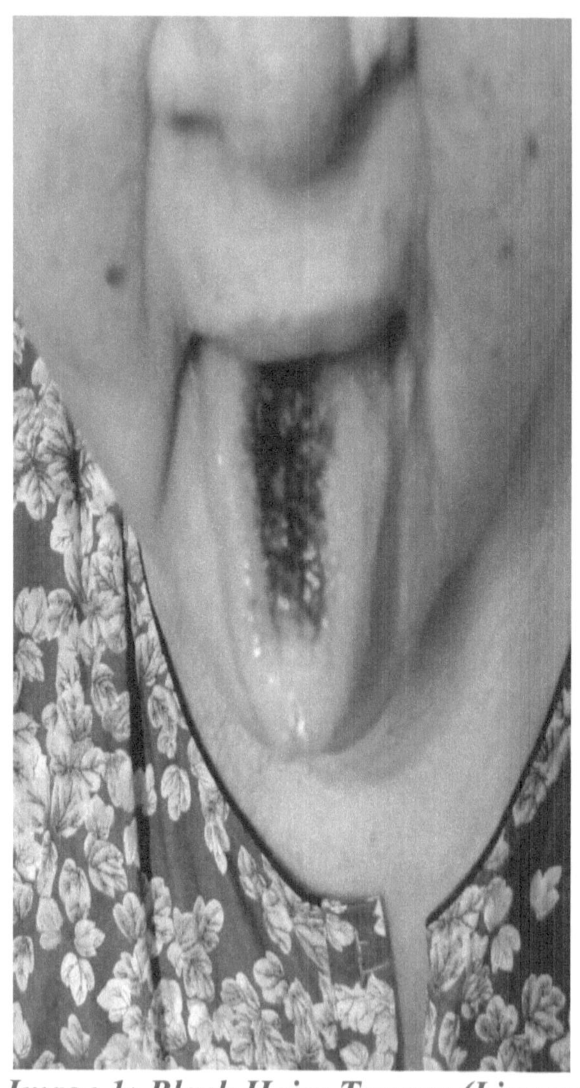

Image 1: Black Hairy Tongue (Lingua Villosa Nigra), Before Treatment Picture

This condition is also known as Black tongue, where the discolouration is due to an accumulation of Keratin on the tongue, the pigment that gives your hair its black colour. This condition may be caused by an overuse of antibiotics or an overgrowth of some bacteria and yeast on the tongue immediately after a long treatment. In this case, it was the overuse of antibiotics.

I could have given Lachesis on the basis of appearance alone. If you take out Kent's repertory and search Tongue, Black, you will find Lachesis to be a well-recognised remedy. Lachesis's action on the whole oral cavity is well known. This, along with the low vitality state, was enough to give Lachesis.

But the prescription was further supported by her symptoms, like aggravation in sleep and intolerance of anything around her neck. All of them, when combined together, were pointing towards Lachesis.

The sleep aggravation part was narrated by her son, who accompanied her, and the intolerance of anything around the neck was the observation.

Despite the cold winter season, I noticed that she is wearing nothing around her head, neck and shoulders. When asked, I got my final confirmatory symptom.

Path to Lachesis :

- Blackish discolouration.
- Sleep aggravation,
- Intolerance of anything around the neck.

Just plain facts. No deep dive into deeper emotional states. By pure observation, you can unearth many unsaid symptoms.

This is a skill that, like any other skill, gets better with time. But only when you allow it to develop. It will never develop if you keep focusing on asking more and more questions. Learn the skill to observe, and I am sure you will master it one day.

Coming back to the case, she recovered

quickly. The discolouration started fading on the first day, and after 7 days, it was gone completely (Please check images 2 and 3).

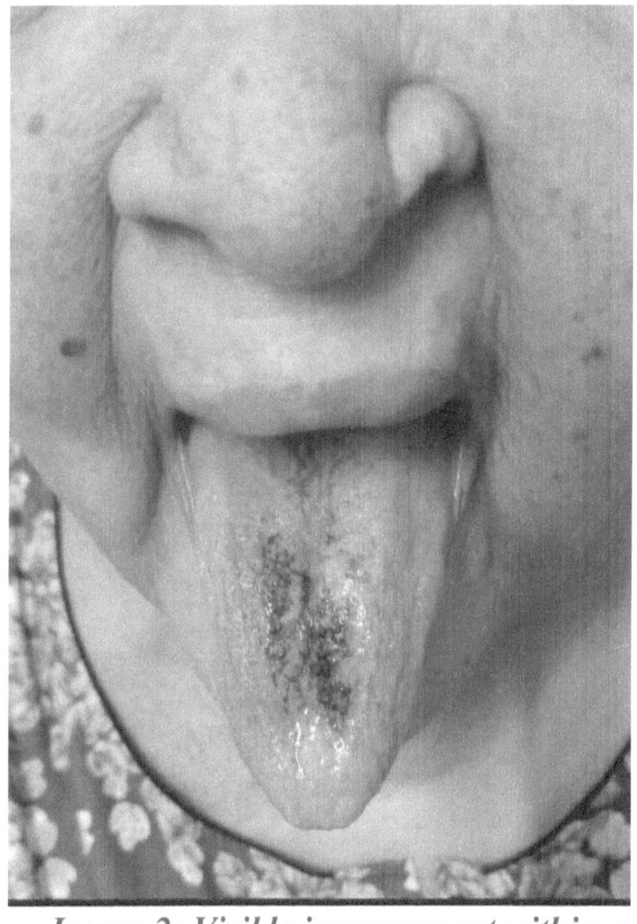

Image 2: Visible improvement within a few hours

Always Remember: 2-3 Strong, fact-based physical symptoms that are clearly evident are way more powerful than a list of 10-15 mental symptoms generated after a long exhaustive case taking.

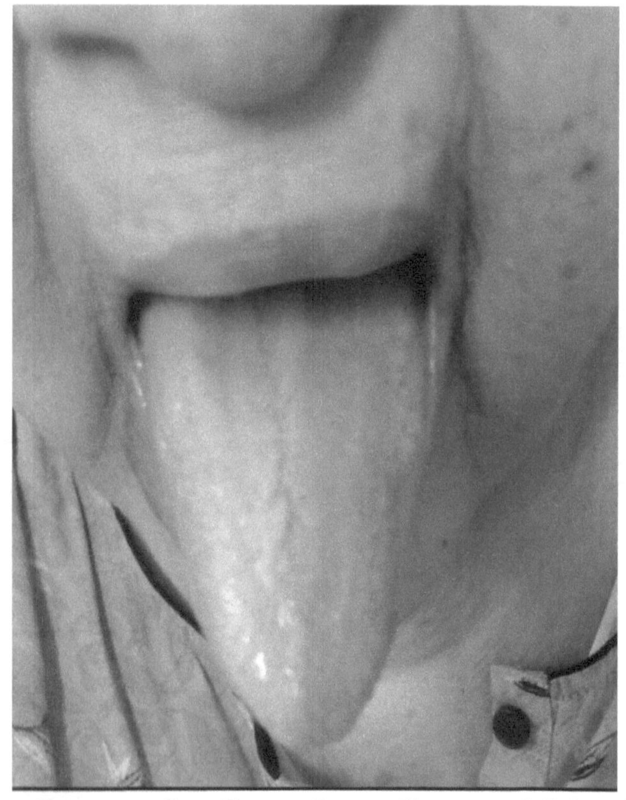

Image 3: Complete Cure within 7 days

It was like a Miracle to everyone. Even the Allopathic Doctors were surprised by such a quick recovery. This is the power of fact-based prescribing. This is the power of Homoeopathy.

CASE NO 2: MIGRAINE

A 50-year-old, graceful woman walked into my clinic, her face etched with quiet suffering. She had been enduring **recurrent migraine headaches** for many years — attacks so intense that they would **paralyse her day-to-day functioning**. But one incident stood out and made her seek deeper healing.

A few days prior, she was travelling in a car with family, heading toward a joyous occasion — a relative's wedding. The day was bright and sunny. As the car moved under the midday sun, she suddenly experienced a **burst of severe headache**, intense and pulsating. The pain hit her like a storm, leaving her unable to mask it anymore.

Despite being in the company of others,

she began to **cry uncontrollably** — something she rarely did, especially in public. The **emotional and physical distress was so overwhelming** that they had to **abort the journey and return home** immediately. She told me that this incident was so embarrassing for her that she decided to consult me as soon as possible.

The way she described those **initial few minutes** — how the pain began, how it escalated, and how she behaved — was enough for me to arrive at the remedy. The essence of her migraine, her emotional reaction, and her silent struggle was unmistakably pointing to **Natrum Muriaticum.**

Here are the **key matching symptoms** that supported my prescription:

1. Migraine Aggravated by Sun

Natrum Mur has one of the most prominent modalities: **Headache triggered or worsened by exposure to sunlight,** especially during or after travel in hot weather.

2. <u>Weeping During Pain, Yet Hating Consolation</u>

She began **crying with the headache**, an emotional overflow, which Natrum Mur is known for. Although she cried, she later admitted she felt worse when others tried to console her — she preferred to be left alone. This combination — **crying with pain** and **aversion to consolation** — is very telling for Natrum Mur.

3. <u>Suppressed Emotions</u>

She was more affected by the **embarrassment of breaking down publicly** than the pain itself. This points to Natrum Mur's **deep emotional reserve**. Natrum Mur patients often suppress grief, hurt, or tears for years until a breaking point arrives, like this migraine attack during a happy event.

Result: She was completely better after 15 days. Her recurrent headaches disappeared and have not returned even once in the last 8 years. This again proves the power of Homoeopathy.

Note: Many of you may feel I'm against using mental symptoms in prescribing. That's not true.

What I'm against is the **forced and fanciful digging** — searching for mental symptoms just to make a case look "deep."

When a mental or emotional state is central to a case, **it doesn't need to be extracted — it presents itself automatically.**

Often, **how and why the patient comes to you already says everything**. The way the case unfolds, the words they use, the emotions they carry — it's all there, right at the surface. **But only if you're paying attention.**

When a mental symptom truly matters, **It walks in with the patient :**

- It breathes through their first few sentences.

- It sits in the silence between their words.
- **How they enter, why they came, how they speak, the pain they carry within themselves.**

That's your materia medica right there, if only you listen.

The remedy lies not in what you dig out with effort but in what stands out effortlessly.

We don't need to search in the shadows when the light is already pointing at the remedy.

CHAPTER 7

Miracles in Moments: A Gallery of Transformations

There are times when words fall short, and the result speaks louder than any detailed case history. This chapter is a celebration of such moments. No elaborate narratives, no complex rubric analysis, no emotional excavations. Just raw, undeniable healing captured in still frames. These before-and-after images are not just photographs—they are turning points. They reveal what miracles are possible with Homoeopathy.

Each transformation you see here was achieved not through lengthy consultations or deep dives into past traumas but through simple, fact-based Homoeopathy. Let these silent visuals remind us: When you listen to the body, it whispers the remedy.

Please note: I have intentionally chosen

not to disclose the names of the remedies used in these cases. This is not to withhold information but to avoid any temptation toward self-prescribing, which can often be misleading or harmful without proper understanding. These cases are not shared as 'recipes' but as evidence of what is possible when Homoeopathy is practised with clarity, respect for facts, and deep clinical insight.

While I've shared exact remedies in a few earlier cases for educational purposes, I've chosen not to do so here, for a reason. This sacred science must not be reduced to a Google search for shortcuts. Each cure you see here is the result of deep listening, sharp observation, and a remedy chosen with respect to the *actual clinical condition* presented. These images are meant to inspire belief in what is *possible* with Homoeopathy, not to encourage untrained individuals to self-prescribe. Healing is an art, and it deserves to be practised with both precision and responsibility.

CASE OF GALL BLADDER STONES

Gall bladder stones are often dismissed as surgical cases—even by fellow Homoeopaths. "Kidney stones, yes. But GB stones? Not possible," they say.

While kidney stones often pass out of the system within 2–3 days of correct homoeopathic treatment, gallbladder stones demand more time and patience. But that doesn't make them incurable. The belief that gallbladder stones must be operated on is outdated and limiting. With accurate, fact-based Homoeopathy, even gallbladder stones can dissolve over time—gently, naturally, and without a knife.

This case proved exactly that. Two stones in the Gall bladder, both 5.5 mm, are clearly seen on the ultrasound. The patient was advised to undergo surgery by allopathic doctors. But with just three months of correct homoeopathic treatment, both stones completely disappeared. No surgery. No hospital. Just solid, focused prescribing. It's time we stop doubting our own system. Homoeopathy works—when done right.

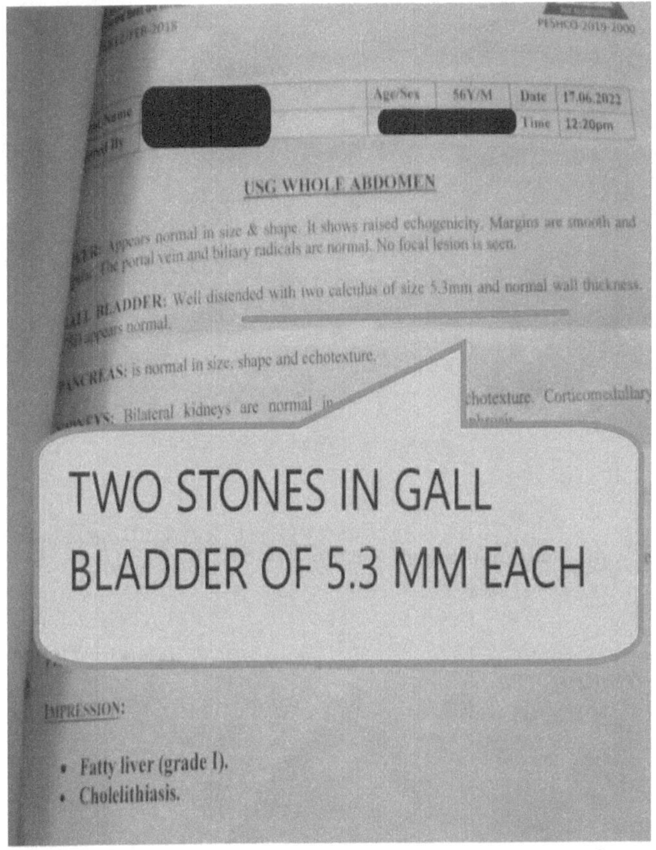

Image 4: Two Gall Bladder stones of 5.5 mm each (Patient's name hidden due to privacy reasons)

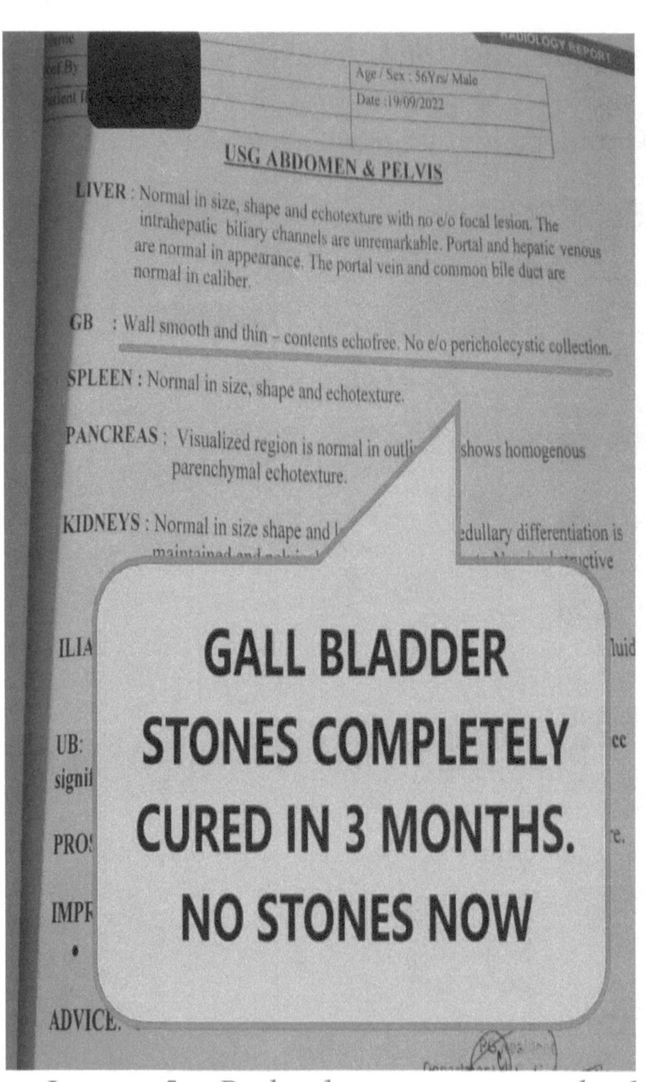

Image 5: Both the stones completely dissolved after just 3 months of treatment

CASES OF HYPOTHYROIDISM

It's widely believed that once diagnosed with **hypothyroidism**, you're destined to take thyroid supplements for life. But **Homoeopathy tells a different story**—a story of hope, healing, and real possibility.

These images show something simple yet powerful—**TSH levels reducing gradually and naturally** with fact based Homeopathic treatment.

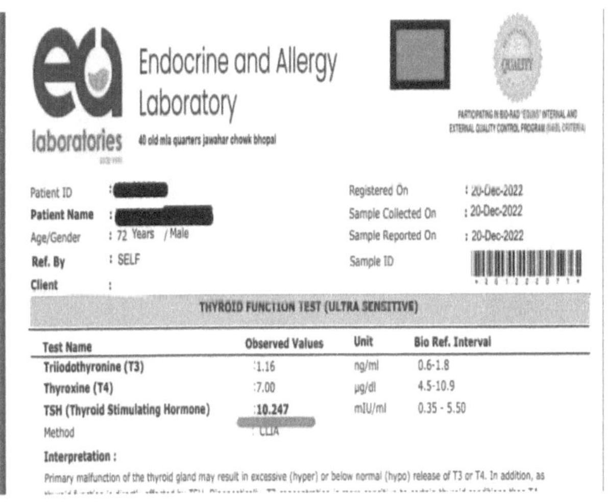

Image 6: TSH LEVEL 10.247, HYPOTHYROIDISM

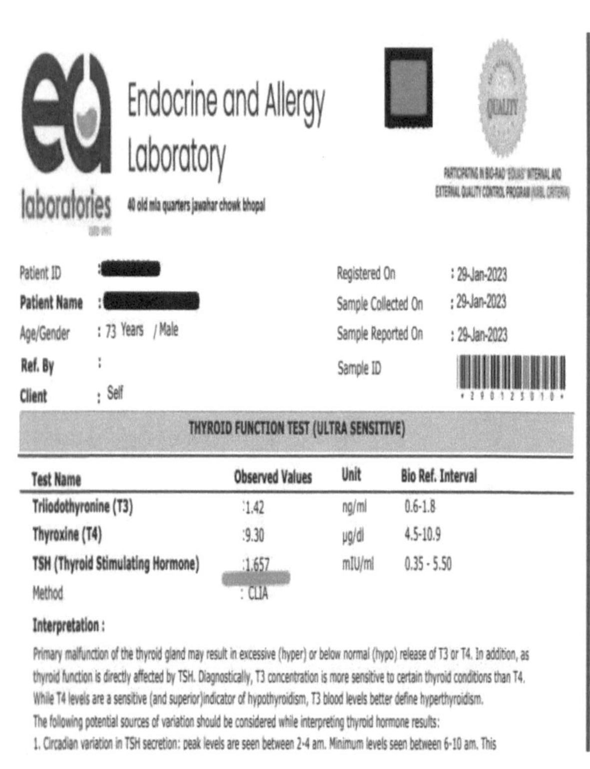

THYROID FUNCTION TEST (ULTRA SENSITIVE)			
Test Name	Observed Values	Unit	Bio Ref. Interval
Triiodothyronine (T3)	:1.42	ng/ml	0.6-1.8
Thyroxine (T4)	:9.30	µg/dl	4.5-10.9
TSH (Thyroid Stimulating Hormone)	:1.657	mIU/ml	0.35 - 5.50
Method	: CLIA		

*Image 7: **TSH CAME DOWN FROM 10 TO 1.657 WITHIN ONE MONTH***

The reduction of TSH from 10.24 to 1.65 in only one month, with only Homoeopathic medicines, proves that Homoeopathy works in Thyroid cases too.

Sharing a few more Hypothyroid cases

where Homoeopathy brought down the TSH levels with marked improvement in the patient's overall well-being, symptomatology and vitality.

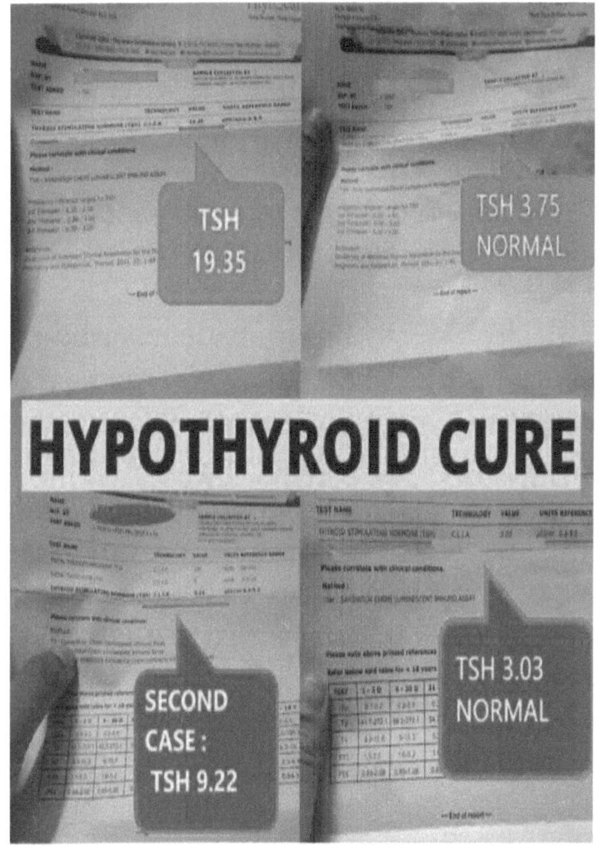

Image 8 A FEW MORE CASES OF COMPLETE HYPOTHYROID CURE

CASES OF BENIGN PROSTATIC HYPERTROPHY (BPH OR PROSTATOMEGALY)

The following cases stand as proof that not every enlarged prostate needs a scalpel.

With carefully selected Homoeopathic treatment, the prostate size reduced significantly, easing symptoms and restoring comfort, without surgical intervention.

I have seen many patients who were advised surgery for their enlarged prostate years back, and now they are living a normal life. It wasn't overnight, but it was real and repeatable. Imagine the blessings these patients gave to Homoeopathic science. When you bring down their main fear (yes, fear of Prostate cancer is real in all BPH patients), you are not only treating a condition; you are healing a soul. You are healing their fears.

Now sharing a few cases where the Prostate was enlarged and the patient was advised surgery, but they recovered completely under Homoeopathic medicines.

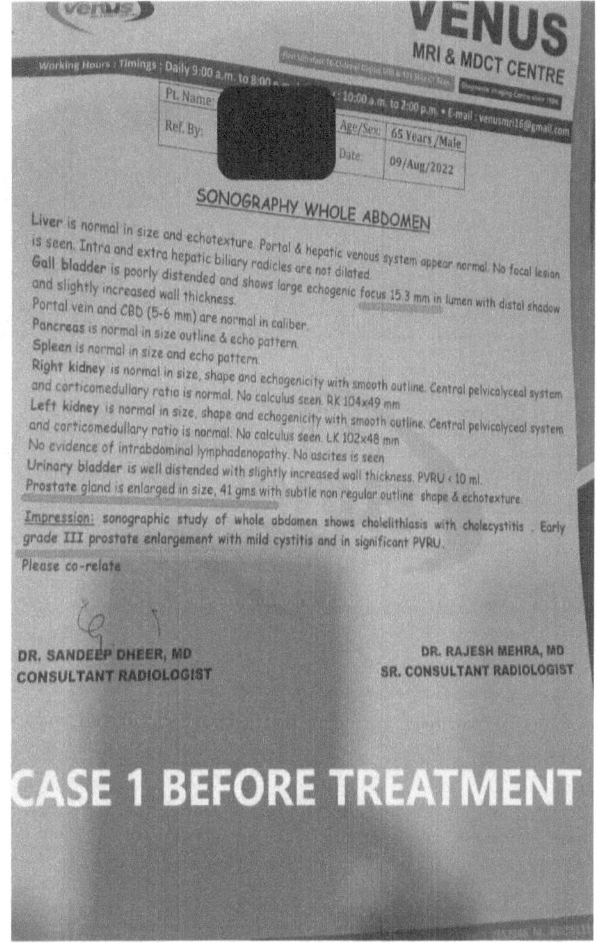

Image 9: CASE 1 OF BPH, PROSTATE ENLARGED, SIZE 41 GMS

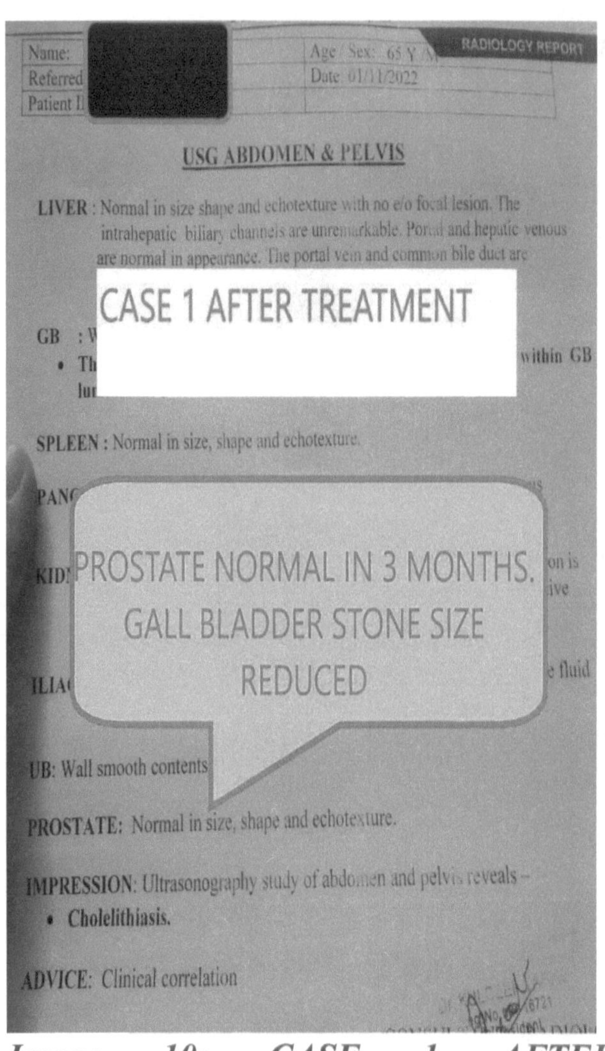

Image 10: CASE 1 AFTER TREATMENT, PROSTATE SIZE NORMAL, SURGERY AVOIDED

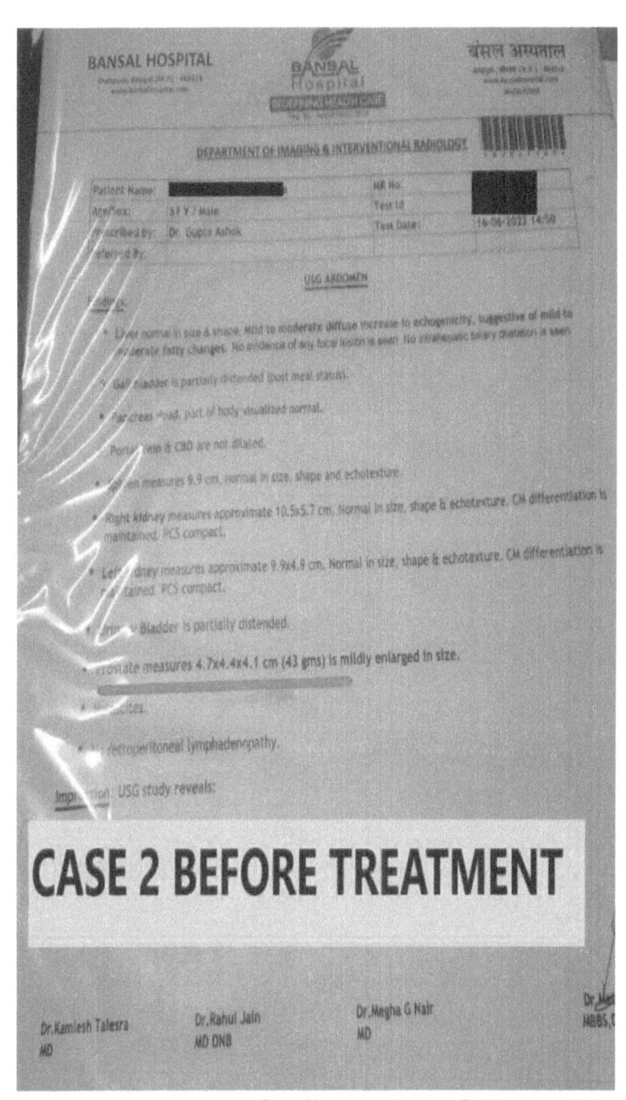

Image 11: CASE 2 OF BPH, ENLARGED PROSTATE, SIZE 43 GMS

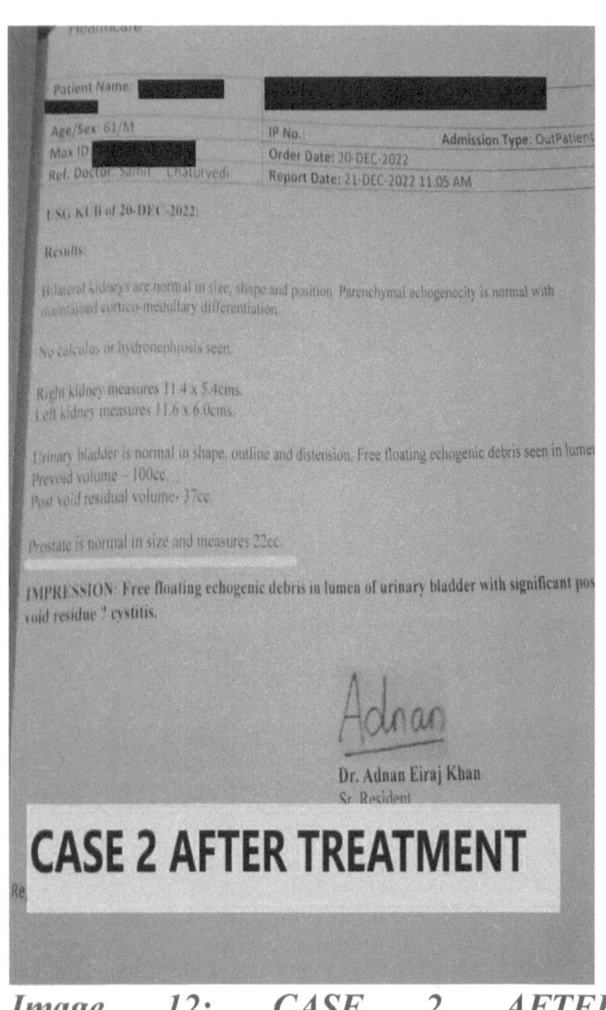

Image 12: CASE 2 AFTER HOMOEOPATHIC TREATMENT, PROSTATE SIZE RETURNED TO NORMAL (NORMAL SIZE 22-24 GMS).

THREAT OF HIGH PSA

When a patient is diagnosed with an enlarged prostate, the first step is often a PSA (Prostate-Specific Antigen) test to rule out the possibility of prostate cancer. If the PSA level is elevated beyond the normal range (0–4), a prostate biopsy is commonly recommended to exclude malignancy.

It is widely believed that as long as PSA levels remain high, the risk of the prostate enlargement turning cancerous also remains significant.

With the correct homoeopathic treatment, we have not only been able to **bring PSA levels back to normal**, but more importantly, **we provide the patient with immense mental relief**—relief from the constant fear of a lurking cancer diagnosis, from that invisible sword hanging over their head.

This healing is not just physiological. It is psychological, emotional, and deeply human. Sharing below the before and after pics of a case where PSA came back to normal with

Homoeopathic medicines alone, providing immense mental relief to the patient.

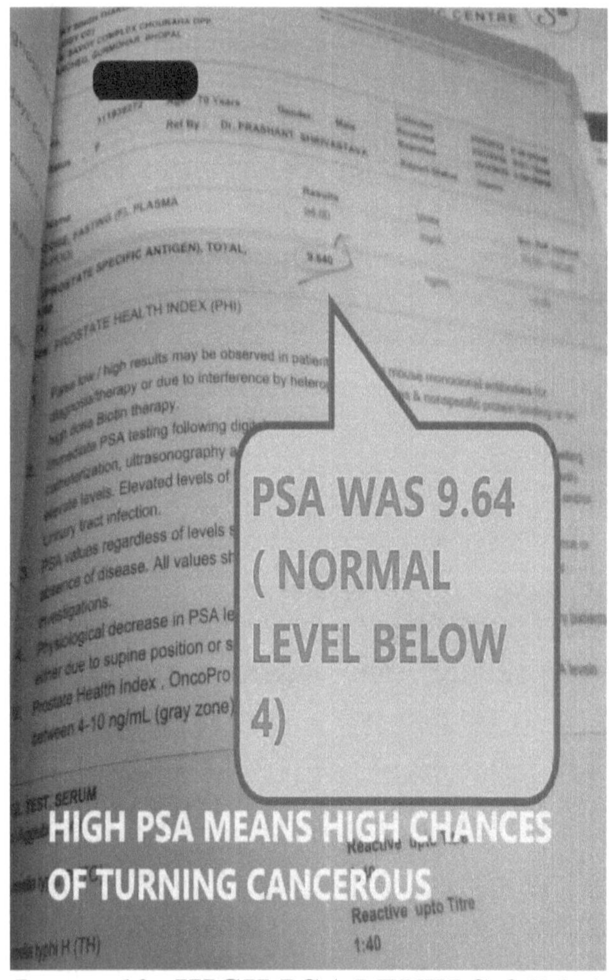

Image 13: HIGH PSA LEVELS OF 9.4

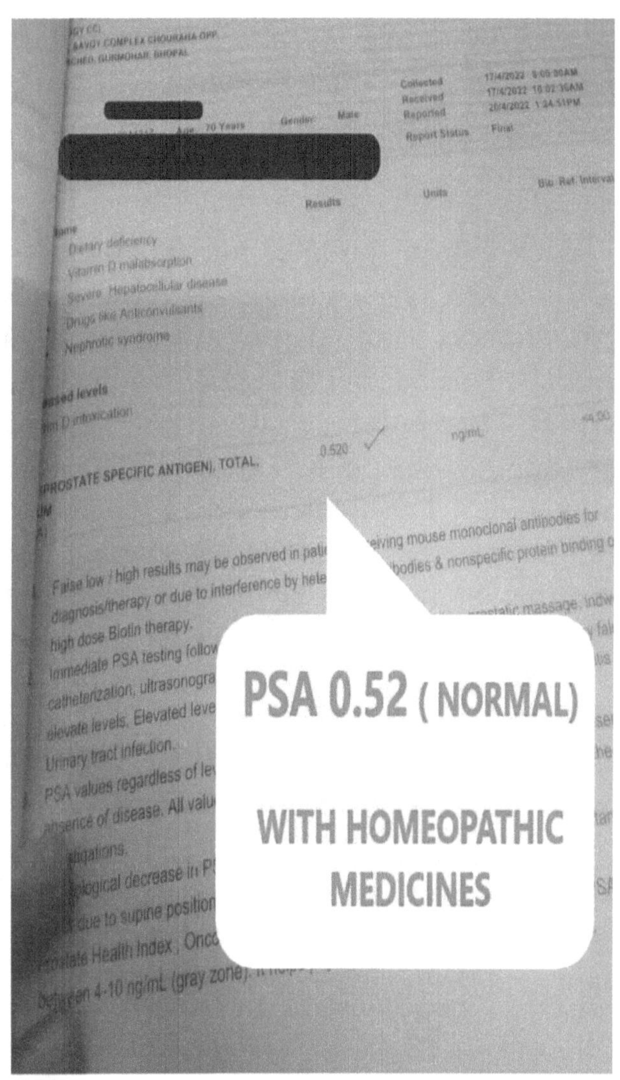

Image 14:PSA BACK TO NORMAL WITH HOMOEOPATHIC MEDICINES

As you've journeyed through this visual gallery, you've witnessed what words alone often fail to express—**that transformation is not just a possibility, but a reality**.

Each before-and-after image tells a story that modern science might call **"incurable,"** but Homoeopathy dared to question that verdict. This chapter is a quiet revolution—**a visual reminder that what appears unchangeable can begin to shift.** Sometimes, the medicine is in the method. But most times, it's in the unwavering belief that the impossible is simply the unexplored.

So the next time someone tells you, "This can't be cured," **don't just accept it as the final word**. Seek out a skilled Homoeopath near you—**because you might just be pleasantly surprised by what Homoeopathy can bring to the table.** Often, the cure you're told doesn't exist is simply one you haven't yet explored.

CHAPTER - 8

IMPOSSIBLE IS A MYTH

Until 1954, it was universally believed that no human being could run a mile in under four minutes. Coaches, athletes, scientists—even medical experts—agreed that it was physically impossible. But then came Roger Bannister. On May 6, 1954, he ran the mile in 3 minutes and 59.4 seconds—and shattered the illusion of impossibility. What's more fascinating? Just weeks later, others started breaking the same barrier. What had changed? The human body? No. The human belief.

The same principle applies to healing. Until someone cures a case labelled as 'incurable,' it remains in the realm of fantasy. But the moment it's done once—correctly, clearly, confidently—it becomes a reference point for the rest of the world. This book is full of such moments. Each case is not just a cure—it is a declaration that **impossible is**

simply something not yet done. The moment one person does it, the door opens for others.

We often confuse **ignorance with impossibility**. Just because we don't know how something works, we label it as unworkable. But It feels impossible until we figure out how to do it; just like Roger Bannister broke the 4-minute mile barrier when the entire world believed it couldn't be done. Once he did it, dozens followed. **The barrier wasn't physical—it was mental.** It just needed one person to show the way.

When you read about a black discoloured tongue that cleared up completely without antifungals...

When you witness a chronic migraine vanishing with one dose of the correct remedy...

When gall bladder stones, previously destined for surgery, dissolve quietly over three months...

When eruptions, pigmentation, and bleeding disorders reverse before your eyes...

When Surgical cases like Benign Prostatic enlargement and Renal Calculi get a complete cure....

It shakes you. And then it shifts you.

Apart from the cure itself, it also shakes the popular belief that to get such remarkable results, one needs to undergo a three-hour-long marathon case taking. That belief gets shattered, too.

All these cases weren't cured by long theoretical speeches or endless mental probing. They were healed through simple, sharp, observation-based prescribing. Sometimes within 5-10 minutes.

Sometimes, just one word from the patient unlocked the remedy. These are **not tales of luck**—they are proof of what's possible when you truly understand the art and science of Homoeopathy.

What was once considered a miracle is now a method.

What was dismissed as an anecdote is now evidence.

What was labelled "incurable" now quietly walks out of clinics, smiling.

This book is not just a collection of cases—**it's a doorway**, a glimpse into a realm where Homoeopathy isn't slow, vague, or theoretical but rapid, precise, and deeply real.

A Note to My Fellow Homoeopaths

To each one of you walking this noble path, I want to say—**yes, it's possible.**

What looks extraordinary today can become routine tomorrow if you only trust your training, senses, and inner voice. You don't need 3-hour marathons. You don't need to drown in theories. You need clarity, courage, and consistency.

If I could do it, **you can do it too**.

I wasn't born with a magic wand. I just believed that Homoeopathy works, even when the world laughed. I learned to observe deeply, think simply, and **trust the facts in front of me more than the doubts in my mind.**

And you—yes, you- can do even better.

Keep going. Keep healing. Keep believing.

Because the world needs more miracle-workers who are quietly, fearlessly, **making the impossible happen** every day.

If this book gave you even a small spark, a moment of inspiration, or a deeper belief in our beautiful science, I would be deeply grateful if you could leave a short review. Your words will not just support this work, but may be the reason another Homoeopath dares to believe in themselves.

With warmth, faith, and respect,

Dr. Jayesh Shah,

M.D (Hom), Mumbai.

www.ingramcontent.com/pod-product-compliance
Lightning Source LLC
Chambersburg PA
CBHW031445150726
47990CB00007B/2619